Generational Emotional Mapping

Gravitational Functional Mapping

Generational Emotional Mapping

Reprogramming the Subconscious with Essential Oils

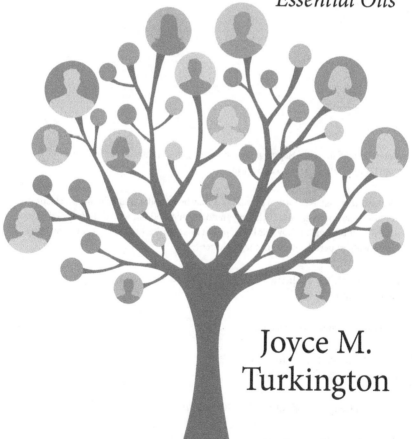

Joyce M.
Turkington

K-BAY PUBLICATIONS
Homer, Alaska

Published by K-Bay Publications
Homer, Alaska

Cover Image: iStock.com/anamad

ISBN: 978-0-9993178-0-8 (paperback)
ISBN: 978-0-9993178-1-5 (e-book)

Library of Congress Control Number: 2017912620

First K-Bay Publications printing: September 2017

Table of Contents

Acknowledgment

First and foremost, I want to give credit to God and my Savior Jesus Christ for lifting me up through years of discovery. In my loneliest and darkest hours of doubt and discouragement, when I've felt all alone on this journey, they have never failed me. They've always sent angels to lift me up and guide me to the next level.

Special thanks to my husband Alan. You have been my rock; you are the glue that held it all together.

Thank you, Shirley and Sharon, for your friendship and support during the months and years of education and working together to build a business.

To our guys—Dave, Alan, and Ron: Thank you for your support, your hours spent building and remodeling, encouraging, and funding us.

To my children, Joy, Scott, Treva, and Matthew: I love you to the moon and back. Thank you for putting up with all my crazy ideas.

Thank you, Nylah; you are a godsend to me and this work.

Stephanie, thanks for introducing me to these amazing oils, for your patience in getting me to finally try them and then for traveling all the way to Alaska to educate me.

To my clients who have also been my teachers, and to the brave souls who took the G.E.M. Therapy Training: thank you for sharing how it has blessed your lives and that of your families.

To Karol Truman: thank you for paving the way and taking the time to mentor me and share your insight with me. This book would not be the powerful tool it is today without your pioneering spirit in the field of Energy Healing.

To my brother Jim, and my dear friend Nancy: thank you for always being there for me, listening to my ideas and dreams, and for never telling me I was losing it.

To those I know I have forgotten to mention by name: thank you all for your support and encouragement.

Finally, thank you to my dear sweet mother who always believed in me.

Thank you all from the bottom of my heart.

Disclaimer

ATTENTION

If you are experiencing medical issues, you need to contact your doctor for treatment. This book is not meant to take the place of medical care. Aromatherapy has been shown to assist the body by helping to lessen the stress of daily living. When stress is reduced, the body is better able to deal with acute illness.

The Protocol discussed in this book is the result of my years of study and application of different energy healing modalities. This work is spiritual in nature but not meant to be religious. I have worked with people from all religions and walks of life. I have worked with individuals who don't hold any religious beliefs. Over the years I have always looked for truth that supports health and wellbeing, regardless of what or with whom I was studying. Through this whole process I stay true to my core beliefs. I would hope you would be able to do the same as you read and implement this work. I hope that you will feel free to adapt or adjust words or concepts to be in alignment with yours.

Introduction

In my mid-twenties, I was diagnosed with multiple sclerosis (MS). Over the years I tried many things to address the symptoms of MS. I asked for a blessing of healing from the elders of our church. In the blessing, I was told that if I did the things the Lord required of me, I would be fine. I can remember thinking to myself that I didn't know what "fine" was according to God. I could be fine in a wheelchair, I could be fine up and walking around, or I could be fine dead. I decided that I would just do the best I could at being a good, caring, compassionate person. However, I wasn't going to lie down for MS.

In 1970 there wasn't much to offer in the way of medicine to treat my condition. My family physician, Dr. Enebo, suggested that I go and visit with Dorothy, a lady in our town who had lived with MS most of her adult life and seemed to be doing well. So, I made contact and spent some time with Dorothy, learning all the things she had experienced over the years concerning supplements, vitamins, minerals, diet, etc., to ease the discomfort of the disease. When I left, I felt encouraged for the first time in months. I began to incorporate the vitamins and supplements she found to be beneficial. To my delight I began to see an improvement in my MS symptoms. I was focusing on vitamins and supplements, working to lessen my stress, and cleaning up my diet.

Years later, I went back to school and became a licensed certified nutritionist in 1995. During my schooling, I had to study many alternative therapies, including electrodermal screening (computerized energy testing) and homeopathy. I was already somewhat familiar with homeopathy as I had used homeopathic medicine with my family for many years.

In 1998, I opened my practice in nutrition. During this time, I investigated many different modalities of healing, some more helpful than others. My desire was to become familiar with the many different therapies available in my community so I could speak from experience when recommending different options to my clients. I experimented with Emotional Freedom Technique (EFT), Reiki, Neuro-emotional Technique (NET), Healing Touch, and of course, homeopathy. I experienced relief from my symptoms with most of these therapies; however, homeopathy seemed to provide the most. As a practitioner, I wasn't interested in chasing and treating symptoms; rather, I wanted to get to the root of the issue. Being a student of homeopathy I learned that familial patterns were part of the history that helped the homeopath decide what remedy to give. One aspect of a patient's symptoms is the mind, or how one feels, thinks, and acts when ill or out of sorts. I found that our emotions and perceptions play a major role in the symptoms being expressed. The homeopath is aware of familial predisposition to various emotions, which play a part in disease. I have always been fascinated with how homeopathic remedies are made and their strengths. I always felt that root emotions were generational in nature. I likened the effects of an emotion with the making of a homeopathic remedy: the more it is diluted (passed on generationally), the stronger it becomes. The following information is from the book *Homeopathic Medicine at Home,* by Maesimund B. Panos, M.D. "The third law of homeopathy, the law of potentization, refers to the preparation of a homeopathic remedy. Each is prepared by a controlled process of successive dilutions alternating with succession (shaking), which may be continued to the point where the resulting medicine contains no molecules of the original substance. These small doses are called potencies; lesser dilutions are known as low potencies and greater dilutions as high potencies. As strange as it may seem, the higher the dilution, when prepared in this manner, the greater the potency of the medicine."[1]

Could this process of dilution effect emotions that have passed from one generation to the next without being resolved? If so, perhaps the emotion and its effect on the body would also become stronger and stronger. As we move into the future of healing and reprogramming, more and more practitioners are addressing generational triggers. The online magazine, *New Scientist,* published an article entitled "Fear of a Smell Can be Passed Down Several Generations." In the body of the piece, in the section subtitled "Brain Change," it talks about experiments with mice and cherry blossoms. The researchers would put cherry blossoms in the cage while shocking the mice. This created fear and anxiety in the mice whenever

---

1 Panos, Maesimund and Meimlich, Jane. *Homeopathic Medicine at Home.* G.P. Putnam's Sons. 1980. Available on Amazon.

they were exposed to acetophenone, the chemical that mimics the smell of cherry blossoms.

The offspring also had more M71 receptors in their brains than did mice born from parents who had not had the smell conditioning and were more sensitive to it. "There was more real estate devoted to this particular odorant receptor, suggesting that there's something in the sperm that is informing or allowing that information to be inherited," Dias says.

DNA sequencing of sperm from the grandfather mice and their sons also revealed epigenetic marks on the gene encoding M71 that weren't seen in control mice.

Female mice conditioned to fear acetophenone also appeared to transmit this "memory" to the next generation, although epigenetic marks on their eggs have not yet been analyzed.[2]

According to Bruce H. Lipton,

the story of epigenetic control is the story of how environmental signals control the activity of genes. It is now clear that the Primacy of DNA chart described earlier is outmoded. The revised scheme of information flow should now be called the "Primacy of the Environment." The new, more sophisticated flow of information in biology starts with an environmental signal, then goes to a regulatory protein and only then goes to DNA, RNA, and the end result, a protein.

---

2 Geddes, Linda. "Fear of a Smell Can be Passed Down Several Generations." *New Scientist*, December 2013. newscientist.com

The science of epigenetics has also made it clear that there are two mechanisms by which organisms pass on hereditary information. Those two mechanisms provide a way for scientist to study both the contribution of nature (genes) and the contribution of nurture (epigenetic mechanisms) in human behavior. If you only focus on the blueprints, as scientists have been doing for decades, the influence of the environment is impossible to fathom (Dennis 2003; Chakravarti and Little 2003). [3]

In 2004, I began developing a protocol called Genetic Energy Mapping (G.E.M.) therapy. It consists of lists of things that can trigger disharmony in mental, emotional and physical bodies.

By using "Body Testing" these triggers can be identified and assessed to determine what elements in a client's emotional background need to be restored or reprogrammed to resolve the disharmony. I have personally experienced healing when using this therapy on myself. Today, in my mid-60s, I have no symptoms of MS, I have no other illnesses, and I am physically healthy. Mentally, emotionally and spiritually, I have never felt better. My wellness journey began in my mid 20s. There is no magic bullet to healing. It takes dedication, perseverance, commitment, and patience. As stated before I have tried many things to help balance my body, mind and spirit. The tools in my tool kit consist of whole foods, no chemicals, exercise on a regular basis, and using a holistic approach to health and wellness. I have utilized allopathic or main stream medicine as needed. I feed my spirit as well as my body everyday

---

3 Lipton, Bruce H. *The Biology of Belief.* Mountain of Love/Elite Books, 2005. Available on Amazon.com.

through prayer and meditation and through building healthy relationships. The use of essential oils is new to me in the past ten years. They are just one more tool to have in your wellness tool kit. They are very powerful in addressing emotional issues.

In the fall of 2010, I was introduced to a high quality therapeutic brand of essential oils by my dear friend Stephanie Fritz, author of *Essential Oils for Pregnancy, Birth & Babies*.[4] Little did I know how that would change my life and the way I helped my clients with generational reprogramming of emotional misconception. I found that when I used the essential oils in conjunction with a G.E.M. session, my clients' results were greatly enhanced. There was an increased feeling of calm, joy, and relief, and physical symptoms were soothed or lessened as well.

As I started using the oils and learning about their aromatic qualities, I created a binder to record the powers of the various essential oils to identify the generational programming that contributes to disharmony and illness, which is the basis of this book. The information on single oils will be common for any source of essential oils. I list all the affirmations of essential oils and the emotions they address and put them in the protocol of G.E.M. Therapy, simplifying the process of identifying the emotions and the oils to address them. In this book you will find the following:

1. Single oils and blend oils in alphabetic order with their healing affirmations

2. A list of the top four emotions addressed with each oil

---

4 Fritz, Stephanie, *Essential Oils for Pregnancy, Birth & Babies*. Gently Born Publications, 2012. Available on Amazon.com.

3. Complementary oils and oils that will blend with them

You will learn two ways to use essential oils to relieve symptoms that may have a generational origin. First, I will show you how to use the information on oils to reprogram generational emotions that are at the root of the symptoms being expressed. Second, I will teach you how to make a personal blend that will support the reprogramming.

Essential oils have aromatic properties that can assist the body in letting go of old traumas. The olfactory system is anatomically connected to the limbic system of the brain. These systems contribute to the function of long-term memory, emotions, the autonomic nervous system, hormones, blood pressure, heart rate, and attention. Emotions are triggered by smell or aroma. This manual is designed to allow you to quickly find the essential oil that will deal with the emotion(s) at the root of the symptoms being expressed. The emotions that trigger symptoms of disharmony in the mental, emotional, and physical body seldom, if ever, originate with us; rather, they have a familial origin.

This book will guide you in finding all the information you need to reprogram old family patterns that have contributed to emotional issues for generations. Through body testing, you will tap into the "hard drive" where this generational information is stored. You will be able to identify the one or more factors being triggered: Error of Thought, Negative Emotions, Negative Words, Lies, or Evil (intent to do harm).

In his book, *The Biology of Belief*, Bruce H. Lipton states that 95% of the time we are working out of the subconscious[5]. Whenever something happens to us, we view it through one of the lenses of the factors mentioned above, and our subconscious goes searching for the origin of the feeling. As we search to identify the emotion that has been triggered, it could be the result of your great-grandma's original emotional response that has now been generationally pro-grammed into your DNA. When an emotion is based on one or more of the above-listed factors, it isn't based on truth and our body will start to build up or break down tissue to match the in-correct perception that is now running.[6] This creates disharmony in the mind, body, and spirit. Your symptoms could be your early warning system. For example, a generational program of the belief that "there is no sweetness in life" [7] might get triggered. The mes-sage is sent to the pancreas, which processes the sugar in the body. This message, left running long enough, will start to reprogram how the body processes sugar. Lipton states in *The Biology of Belief*, that "[t]he science revealed in this book defines how beliefs control behavior and gene activity, and consequently the unfolding of our lives. The chapter on Conscious Parenting describes how most of us unavoidably acquired limiting or self-sabotaging beliefs that were downloaded into our subconscious minds when we were children."[8]

---

5 Lipton, Bruce H., Ph.D., *The Biology of Belief*, Mountain of Love/Elite Books, 2005. Available on Amazon.com.

6 Hamer, Ryke Geerd. *Summary of The New Medicine*. Overall Productions, August 2000, Available on Amazon.com.

7 Hay, Louise L. *You Can Heal Your Life*. Hay House, 2004. Available on Amazon.com.

8 Lipton, Bruce H., Ph.D., *The Biology of Belief*, Mountain of Love/Elite Books, 2005. Available on Amazon.com.

Chapter 1

What Is Generational Emotional Mapping?

Generational Emotional Mapping Therapy is based on the premises that whenever there is a shock or trauma that is not resolved, the feelings associated with the trauma can be felt in the body, such as an aching heart, a knot in the stomach, etc. These feelings become associated with emotions. These emotions can have a direct effect on our well-being if left unresolved. G.E.M. Therapy recreates a map of where it began, with whom it started with, what factor the emotion is running through, the oil that will address the emotion(s) and the affirmation of the oil to create a shift in the old incorrect perception. This information is all held in the subconscious energetic body or the physical body and can be accessed with body testing (a form of kinesiology).

When I became interested in energy healing I was introduced to computer models of testing the body and it was very fast and efficient. The computer had a list of items that would be presented to the body in a grid form, through biofeedback. The body would quickly break the list down by assessing the grid for a matching frequency. The computer could break the grid down from top to bottom through a process of elimination to identify a vitamin, remedy, supplement, etc. My desire was to allow a person to process in the same way without the computer by numbering everything that was to be tested. I found that once you made the list and numbered it you didn't have to read the statements or items in the list—all you had to do was affirm, "The root oil is in Column 1-6." Once you have identified the Column you would then find the Essential Oil in that Column. With this numbering system, I could now process large amounts of information very quickly. I knew from years of study and observation that disharmony in my mind, body, and spirit did not always begin with me. Again, the writings of others seem to support my idea that when our thoughts become distorted by an incorrect perception there is the possibility for the function of our body and mind to be effected in a negative way. Consider Bruce H. Lipton's reference to epigenetics:

> Think of the pattern of the test screen as the pattern encoded by a given gene, say the one for brown eyes. The dials and switches of the TV fine-tune the test screen by allowing you to turn it on and off and modulate a number of characteristics, including color, hue, contrast, brightness, vertical and horizontal holds. By adjusting the dials, you can alter the appearance of the pattern on the screen, while not actually changing the original broadcast pattern. This is precisely the role of regulatory proteins. Studies of protein synthesis reveal that epigenetic 'dials' can create 2,000 or more variations of proteins of the same gene blueprint [Bray 2003; Schmuker, et al, 2000] . . . In this

epigenetic analogy, the test pattern on the screen represents the protein backbone pattern encoded by a gene. While the TV's controls can change the appearance of the pattern they do not change the original pattern of the broadcast (i.e. the gene). Epigenetic control modifies the read-out of the gene without changing the DNA code. He talks about this change in pattern can turn a gene on or turn it off, there by changing the outcome of the expression of the cells. The epigenetic evidence has become so compelling that some brave scientists are even invoking the "L" word for Jean Baptiste de Lamarck, the much-scorned evolutionist, who believed that traits acquired as a result of environmental influence could be passed on. Philosopher Eva Jablonka and biologist Marion Lamb wrote in their 1995 book *Epigenetic Inheritance and Evolution: The Lamarckian Dimension*, "In recent years, molecular biology has shown that the genome is far more fluid and responsive to the environment than previously supposed. It has also shown that information can be transmitted to descendants in ways other than through the base sequence of DNA."[1]

I began gathering things that I found to be triggers for myself and others who I worked with in my clinic. I found that the "I'm not good enough" belief didn't begin with me because I could also see that belief pattern in my father and his parents or my mother and her parents. I also observed through the computer model that my body had a vast amount of information which I had no conscious knowledge of. What else was in my body computer that could be accessed? As I experimented with body testing, my body would

---

1 Ibid.

identify, if an emotion was generational coming through my father or my mother or both. From a list of statements or emotions body testing would identify what was associated with the symptom or issue. Many times, as I gathered this information I would feel the emotions very strongly in my body and mind. At times, I would start crying or get emotional, however it didn't feel like it was mine. It was as if my body was reacting to the emotion and my mind was witnessing the event. I felt I had access to a generational database .

I would like to relate an experience that I had during this time of study, research, pondering and experimenting:

It was a beautiful Sunday. I was sitting in church with my mother, husband and three of our four children. Suddenly my shoulder felt like it was being pulled out of the socket, and pain was shooting down my arm. Because of my study of generational emotions, I started testing with a form of muscle testing using my fingers (I will explain more later). I first checked if the emotion behind pain was mine; it wasn't. I checked for my mom, husband, children, etc., and when the thought of my father popped into my mind, I got a "yes" response that it was an emotion coming through my father. Then I started testing for the actual emotion or negative belief that was running in the background. I was checking things like, fear, anger, anxiety, worthlessness, etc., and when I used the statement, "not good enough" I got a "yes," and I could suddenly see my father in my mind's eye. He was standing with his arms pinned to his side with a big purple rubber band around his middle, and across the band, in bold black letters, were the words "NOT GOOD ENOUGH." Bound behind him in a line was his mother and father and their mothers and fathers and so on as far as the eye could see. They were all looking at me! I was overwhelmed with the feeling of them being stuck and wanting me to help them. I said a silent prayer. "Lord, I don't know who bought into this lie that we aren't good enough. We are all worthy of your love and abundance. Please heal this lie, bringing it forward through time and eternity from whom it started to me. Heal every aspect and incorrect perception, lie and misgiving through all generations of time. Amen." At that very instant the band exploded into a million pieces and everyone moved away, going in different directions and the pain in my shoulder was gone. My mother leaned over and whispered, "What was that all about?" "Oh, it was just Dad," I whispered back. Mother said, "He never comes to me like that." It was as if I heard my father's voice in my mind saying. "Because you take the time to listen."

This experience was very profound for me. It was so real, it was like it was etched in my mind in techno color and stereo sound. I came away with the insight that an emotion could have its origin farther back than I had imagined. I also learned the following:

1. That negative emotions or beliefs can "bind" us up and hinder movement. (Purple Band)

2. That the emotion showed up in my physical body. (the pain in my shoulder)

3. That I had the power to bring attention to the situation by gathering information from the generational database and speak words of healing.

4. That my words energetically exploded the band and the physical pain stopped.

Maybe it was just mind over matter, perhaps just acknowledging that "we are all good enough" shifted my "dials" to be in focus. In any event, I was off and running with this new insight. I made list after list of things that affect and infect us, that trigger us, and that heal us, and I added them to my binder. I had no idea what to call this information. It helped me identify who experienced the root emotion that was being passed forward, what the emotion was, who it began with, the belief or negative statement, and then blessing or asking for healing. I could use this formula to get to the root of the symptoms being expressed and I experienced amazing results, as well as my clients.

I attended a conference that featured Bruce Lipton, in Clearwater, Florida. He spoke about generational subconscious programs that are passed from generation to generation and that those programs needed to be discovered and reprogrammed. He spoke of energy psychology (EP), which is a collection of mind-body approaches for understanding and improving human functioning. EP focuses on the relationship between thoughts, emotions, sensations, and behaviors, and known bioenergy systems (such as meridians and the biofield). Everyone at the conference was buzzing over how to do this and I was sitting there looking at the workbook in my lap, with lists of triggers, factors, phases of existence, healing statements, and power words. I knew that over the past three years of gathering information, affirming, and having friends and family be my testers, I had come upon something that was beyond me. I could have never created something as detailed and intricate as this on my own. It was inspiring that with all my hours of study, research, pondering, meditation and experimenting, I had been led to the same conclusion as this doctor. He was presenting the science behind the ideas that I had based on my personal experiences.

As I sat there pondering this revelation, I saw this process of discovery as following a treasure map, picking up clues along the way to find the "treasure," i.e., the top triggers at the root of the generational programming, and then being able to change the perception. These triggers had the possibility of resonating from previous generations. They were now energy memories begging to be healed. The person who first experienced these triggered emotions, and the place and time, are long gone, but the memory of the smell, sight, touch, sound, time, and place along with a thousand other triggers were imprinted in the body's DNA and transferred to the tissues.

Karol Truman, in her book *Feelings Buried Alive Never Die*, stated: "Changing the way we THINK by changing the way we FEEL is faster, much more effective, and further reaching."[2] This means that if we can identify the feeling that created the thought which caused the action or emotion, we will have better results.

Challenges are part of life. They serve to refine and build us so that we can learn to be leaders and champions for good. Life experiences are most often registered through the lenses of Error of Thought, Negative Emotions, Negative Words, Lies or Evil (Intent to do Harm.) That day in Florida, I came up with the name of Genetic Energy Mapping. The more I worked with emotions, I reframed it to be Generational Emotional Mapping or G.E.M. therapy.

---

2 Truman, Karol K. *Feelings Buried Alive Never Die*. Revised edition. Olympus Distributing, 1991. Available on Amazon.com.

Chapter 2

Body Testing

*I*n his book, *Power VS. Force*, David R. Hawkins writes the following:

> In 1971, three physiotherapists published a definitive study on muscle testing. Dr. George Goodheart of Detroit, Michigan, made a breakthrough discovery that the strength or weakness of every muscle was connected to the health or pathology of a specific corresponding body organ. He was the founder of applied kinesiology and published several manuals on the subject.
>
> Initially, the most striking finding of kinesiology was a clear demonstration that muscles instantly became weak when the body is exposed to harmful stimuli. For instance, if a patient with functional hypoglycemia put sugar on his tongue, upon muscle-testing, the deltoid muscle (the one usually used as an indicator) instantly went weak. Accordingly, it was discovered that substances that were therapeutic to the body made the muscles instantly become strong. Dr. John Diamond, a psychiatrist who began to use kinesiology in diagnosing and treating

psychiatric patients, which he labeled "behavioral kinesiology." While other investigators were researching the usefulness of the method in detecting allergies, nutritional disorders, and responses to medications, Dr. Diamond used the technique to research the beneficial or adverse effects of a great variety of psychological stimuli, such as art forms, music, facial expressions, voice modulation, and emotional stress . . . his seminars attracted thousands of professionals who returned to their own practices with renewed interest and curiosity as they explored applications of the technique.[1]

To gain a full understanding of kinesiology or muscle-testing, I suggest that you read Hawkins's book, *Power VS. Force.* It is about his twenty years of research and study of this technique.

Over the years different methods have been developed to test the body's response to stimuli. I use the "heel/toe" method of body testing in my clinic. When you make a statement feeling the body weight shift to the toes equals a YES response. If you feel the body weight shift to the heels this equals a NO response. To introduce your body to this testing method, stand in a comfortable position with feet apart, knees flexed, make the statement, "My name is *(use someone else's name)*." You should feel your body weight shift to the heels indicating, NO. Now make the statement, using your given name, "My name is *(given name)*" You should get a yes response. If you learned body testing by a different method that you are more comfortable with use that. Going forward I will refer to body testing as Affirming. I hope that this will always remind you to make

---

1 Hawkins, David R. *Power VS. Force.* Hay House, 2002. Available on Amazon.com.

statements rather than questions when you are body testing. The body works best by affirming or not affirming a statement by using a yes or no indicator.

Chapter 3

Renewal Process

I have used the term "renewal" in this heading instead of "reprogram." It is important to distinguish the nuanced differences in
meaning between the two words. I went to *Merriam-Webster Dic-
tionary* for definitions.

> **Reprogram:** *to make changes—revise—make anew*
>
> **Renew:** *to make new: restore to freshness, vigor, or perfection, to
> make new spiritually: regenerate*

Years ago, I was at a health conference and a doctor from a
Sloan Kettering Hospital was talking about cancer. He made the
statement that we all had cancer cells, and that the trick was to keep
our vibration or frequency high enough to stay above the cancer,
which has a low vibration. My goal has always been to address those
things that lower our energy vibration. Diet, exercise, lifestyle, emotions and feelings all play a part in that energy shift. In 2014, I ran
across information to validate that statement:

Maintaining an alkaline environment is a key to good health. As our voltage drops below a certain level, we begin to experience fatigue. As the voltage further drops (and thus the pH drops) we become prone to developing health problems. Cancer cells, for example, have a pH of about 6.3 and carry a specific voltage. By knowing that chronic disease is associated with low voltage, one might ask an obvious question; "What is my voltage?" Cells are designed to run at a pH of 7.35 (-20 millivolts) to a pH of 7.45 (-25 millivolts). Cell membranes can achieve a temporary "action potential" of up to -90 millivolts. We heal by making new cells. Making new cells requires -50 millivolts. We get sick when we cannot achieve -50 millivolts and thus cannot make new cells. We are thus stuck in chronic disease. All chronic disease is defined by having low voltage. Chronic disease occurs when voltage drops below -20 millivolts.[1]

In the steps below we are going to use a process of discovery to identify key components of the disharmony that is producing either an overabundance of energy that wears things out, or low energy that contributes to an environment for issues to occur in our mental, emotional or physical state. The goal is to bring to our conscious mind the old feelings, thoughts and beliefs that are running in the background that we are unaware of and that have a generational origin. We want to identify those and renew or restore the energy field with truth which will rewrite our programming, allowing for

1 Torres, Marco. *Healing Is Voltage, Prevent Disease*, Web. July 2, 2014. Accessed June 28, 2017. http://preventdisease.com/news/14/070214_Healing-Is-Voltage.shtml

regeneration of the energy field that supports the physical, mental, emotional and spiritual states.

I wrote statements that clarify how we are doing with different issues. You can affirm each statement to see if your programing is in harmony with that statement. As you affirm each statement you should get a yes response. If you get a no response you will know that there is a block created by an emotion or an incorrect perception that is indicating just the opposite. For example, if I were double checking whether I had totally reprogrammed the issue of feeling "not good enough," any of the following statements that produce a no response would indicate the need to discover what emotion was running to negate or distort that truth.

I Am Statements

1. I am free to demonstrate life through truth and love, which support my divine blueprint (by letting go of the feeling of "not good enough")

2. I am ready (to let go of "not good enough")

3. I am willing (to let go of "not good enough")

4. I am able (to let go of "not good enough")

5. I am safe (letting go of "not good enough")

6. I am worthy (to let go of "not good enough")

7. I am supported (in letting go of "not good enough")

8. It is healing for others (for me to let go of "not good enough")

9. I have time (to let go of "not good enough")

10. I have energy (to let go of "not good enough")

The goal is to bring the body's energy field into balance, and the physical body will follow suit. Each essential oil has a frequency or vibration that supports a positive affirmation to address negative emotions. Using Affirming you will be able to quickly identify the essential oil that will address the issue by identifying the emotion(s) running in the background and you will also have the affirmation of the oil to help renew the generational subconscious database.

Essential oils and the power of words can help increase our vibration. This renewal of energy will help the body to function optimally. Each body system has an intelligence that is designed to keep each system functioning properly. We are constantly gathering and sifting through data, which is mostly done without the awareness of our conscious mind. As mentioned earlier, many things can distort the gene expression.

In this renewal process, I wanted all aspects of my being to be whole, well, and happy. I have made a list of what I feel makes up the full expression of who we are now. I refer to this list as "Aspects of Self." This list comes from my study of the Bible, chakras, anatomy, physiology, shamans, healers, the spirit realm, and more. Just as I made lists of things that trigger negative emotions, I made a list of what I viewed as different aspects of myself that could be affected. I will calibrate the aspects of self, to see if they are resonating at 100%. It is a way for me to visualize my journey through space and time. These definitions are my creation. They come from a combination of my religious beliefs, spiritual writings, and science and then my own interpretation from experience. I hope that as you read this list you will be able to adjust the definitions if needed to match your beliefs.

Numbers 1–6 are intangible aspects of ourselves. Numbers 7–20 metaphorically represent our physical systems.

1. Original Intelligence: Intelligence without form.

2. Spirit: We were born or took on a spirit body that looks just like the one we have now.

3. Higher Self: The part of us that is in possession of our spiritual contract, the plan we made before we were born.

4. Super-conscious: Encompasses awareness that sees both material reality and the energy and consciousness behind that reality. The superconscious is where true creativity is found.

5. Subconscious: It records everything we do: every activity we engage in, our thoughts about those activities, our likes and dislikes about our daily encounter, and our generational programming. The subconscious has a tremendous influence on how we think and act when in the conscious state.

6. Conscious: Operates during our daily activities and waking hours. It represents a small portion of our awareness.

7. Skeletal: Represents our feelings of being supported in life.

8. Muscular: Facilitates our free movement through life.

9. Nervous system/brain: Provides a flow of communication between all systems of the body.

10. Senses: Support our intuition or knowing, guiding us to make good choices.

11. Endocrine: The communication within, to balance the male/female aspects of self.

12. Blood: Provides a free flow of joy in life.

13. Heart: The center of love for God, self, family, and humanity.

14. Circulation: Provides a path for giving and receiving, love/abundance.

15. Lymphatic: Supports our self-worth and the essentials of life such as love and joy.

16. Respiratory: Gives us ability to take in the goodness of life.

17. Digestion: Provides understanding of the data coming into our systems daily.

18. Urinary: Provides focus, forgiveness, happiness, and trust of people in our lives

19. Reproductive: The center of all creativity.

20. Integumentary: Provides protection for our external and internal body.

As I have calibrated each of these aspects of self, I have found them to be below 100%. This is an indication to me that there is an issue of some kind running in the back ground that is creating a drag on that aspect of my being. I will use the G.E.M. protocol to find an essential oil that will balance that system. If I focus on the system that has the lowest percentage and address its issues it will often balance other systems that are low or at least raise the calibration. This indicates to me that one system can have a negative as well as a positive effect on other systems in the body.

I am reminded of a New Testament scripture from Luke 11:17: "But he, knowing their thoughts, said unto them, every kingdom divided against itself is brought to desolation; and a house divided against a house falleth." I view my body as a kingdom; if it isn't in balance than the different kingdoms (systems or aspects of self) may be at war with one another or just not able to provide the support needed. When a system is out of balance it can and will affect the whole. When this happens, we see depression creep in, low energy, and illness manifest. Our emotional state tends to follow with a negative outlook.

The whole purpose of G.E.M. therapy is to identify key issues that are preventing the body from recovering from a trauma, no matter its origin. We want to identify what needs to be renewed in the energy field which in turn will support the emotional and physical transformation.

In this process the affirmation of the individual oils becomes the basis of your request for healing or resolution to the problem.

For example, let's say that the oil I identify to address my root issue was ginger, which addresses emotions relating to being a victim, feeling powerless, feeling defeated, and feeling blamed. The affirmation of ginger enables me to be fully present, empowering me to take responsibility and to let go of my feeling of being a victim.

It is my belief that each of the words in the affirmation have a vibration, color, frequency, depth, height, length, width, power and authority. I use these words to describe the words in a way that doesn't limit our understanding of all aspects of the energetic power of words in the affirmation. When you repeat the Renewal Script you are appealing to the intelligence of all your aspects to search your database and make corrections to negativity anywhere it is found in the body and/or the energy field.

I would ask for the original power of (<u>essential oil</u>) **ginger,** *(<u>read affirmation</u>)* **to enable me to be fully present, to empower me to take responsibility, and to let go of being a victim.** *Charge this affirmation into the generational energy field from where the incorrect perception started and with whom it started, bringing it forward through all generations of time with its original power and authority, thereby renewing the energy field. Set and run! Thank you.*

Chapter 4

G.E.M. Therapy Protocol

Generational Reprogramming With Essential Oils

*I*n this chapter, you will learn the steps to identify the feelings, thoughts and emotions that have been handed down from generation to generation. We will be working in reverse as our goal is to identify the emotion, so that we can elicit the feeling or emotion that is at the root.

Preparing for a Generational Emotional Mapping session.

1. Find a quiet place to work.

2. Have a surface that is counter height to lay your book on. I have a 30-in. stool in my office to lay a clipboard or my book on.

3. Have something to write with and a clipboard to hold your Processing Protocol. You will be standing to do your body testing to gather your information. I like to hold the clipboard so that I can record my findings while standing.

4. Until you are familiar with the steps, I would recommend that you make a copy of the Processing Protocol so that you can have it available as your guide. If you process often, as I do, it will become second nature.

Step 1: Make a list of your mental, emotional, and physical complaints, and number them. Affirm which is the #1 issue needing to be addressed.

Step 2: Set your intent. What is your desired outcome? (Easing of physical issues, emotional issues, etc.)

Step 3: Determine to what extent this issue is dragging your energy field down, by calibrating each issue. You should have already established your YES/NO responses for body testing. (If not, go back to the chapter on Body Testing.) Your statement would be, "This issue is allowing my energy to resonate above 50%." If your body affirms YES, then increase the percentage until you identify your maximum energy level. If your body affirms NO, then decrease the percentage. Don't be surprised if your energy is in the minus. I have experienced difficult or longstanding issues with a drag of minus 10–20 thousand or more. This will give you a feel for how taxing and difficult this issue has been for you. Once you have your percentage you need to understand where on the generational time track this feeling-thought-emotion was originally set up. I was told many years ago by a naturopathic doctor that the symptoms of disease were expressions of history. Emotions are at the root of all illness, and emotions are passed from generation to generation unresolved (remember all the generations bound by the negative belief of "not good enough"). Science is beginning to show that a feeling may not originate on our personal time track.

Step 4: Affirm in which phase the incorrect perception was started (see Glossary).

Phase 1: Spiritual childhood.
Phase 2: Spiritual adulthood.
Phase 3: The creation of the physical body.
Phase 4: Integration from the spiritual realm into the physical realm.
Phase 5: Earth life
Phase 6: After-life.

Step 5: Affirm with whom the original incorrect perception started. At times, you may affirm more than one source (see Glossary).

1. Universal Family
2. Tribe: mother/father/both
3. Family: mother/father/both
4. Individual: male/female/both/self

Step 6: Affirm which factors are driving the generational misconception. How an event is perceived will make a difference in how we respond to different triggers. More than one of these factors can be part of the problem. You will need to perform the affirming process with all five to find contributing factors. (See Glossary.)

1. Error of Thought
2. Negative Emotions
3. Negative Words
4. Lies
5. Evil (Intent to do harm)

Step 7: Use the Master Oil List to affirm the root essential oil(s). Your statement will be: "The root essential oil is in Column 1." The column will be identified by your YES/NO indicator. You will then state: "The oil in this column is #1, 2, 3, etc." Again, the oil will be identified by the body response of YES/NO. You will repeat Step 7 until you have identified all the oils needed to address your #1 issue. You will know you have gathered all the oils for this issue when you make the affirming statement, "I have gathered all the oils I need for this phase," and the response is YES.

Step 8: Turn to the page(s) containing the description of the oil(s) and affirm which of the emotions relating to each oil are contributing to the issues. You will find each essential oil has its own page. On each page, you will find the affirmation, the four top emotions the oil is addressing, companion oils, the classification of the oil, and other oils that blend well.

Step 9: Affirm that you need other oils listed on the page to address the issue at hand. If YES, affirm which other oils on the page apply. If NO, continue. If you don't identify an oil on that page then process the columns on the master list to identify the oil needed.

Step 10: Affirm where on the body you will apply the essential oils. Common areas would be the crown of the head, thyroid, heart, liver, pancreas, abdomen, kidneys, or adrenal glands. Sometimes there will be an area of concern such as the knee, shoulder, etc.

Step 11: Apply the essential oil to your fingers, rubbing your thumb and fingers together. Breath aroma of oil in deeply and exhale slowly, emptying your lungs, do this a couple of time and then apply the oil on the affirmed area.

Step 12: Read the Renewal Script. *I would ask for the original power of (essential oil), (read affirmation). Charge it into the generational energy field from where the incorrect perception started and with whom it started, bringing it forward through all generations of time with its original power and authority, thereby renewing the energy field. Set and run! Thank you.* Observe and note any impressions, thoughts, sensations, visions, etc., that may be released.

Step 13: Make the statement, "I have resolved this #1 issue more than 30%." If yes, continue to calibrate up; if no, calibrate down to find the percentage addressed. If it isn't addressed 100% you will repeat **Steps 7–13**. Once you have addressed the number one issue 100%, go back to the other issues and determine if their calibrations have increased. You will find that most of them will have improved from addressing the root issue first. Some will even be 100% addressed. If YES, go back to **Step 3** and process the next issue.

Example Processing Worksheet

Step 1:   1. Sleeplessness 2. Indigestion 3. Headaches
4. **Anxiety**

Step 2:   Set intent

Step 3:   -356%

Step 4:   Phase 4

Step 5:   Family: Father

Step 6:   Error of Thought, Lies

Step 7:   Column 4, Number 3—Roman Chamomile

Step 8:   Purposeless, Frustration

Step 9:   No other oil.

Step 10:   Pancreas

Step 11:   Deep breathing of aroma of chosen oils

Step 12:   Apply the oil to pancreas and read Renewal Script

Step 13:   +45% [Repeat **Steps 4–12** until the issue has been
addressed at 100%]

After every session, be sure to drink plenty of water, and rest if you feel tired. You will have moved a ton of energy so you can experience many different sensations, from thirst, fatigue, and sleepiness to exhilaration. Just remember to listen to your body.

The impressive thing about reprogramming issues at the generational level is that the energy shift happens for others in the family as well! I had a funny experience a few years back when I was struggling with sugar. I was literally binging on goodies daily. So I affirmed the "I Am" Statements: I am free to give up sugar, I am ready to give up sugar, I am willing to give up sugar, and so on. I affirmed every statement and got NO for every single one! The number one statement was that "it wasn't safe to give up sugar." So everyday, the "not safe"thought was being triggered and my response was to self-sooth- by eating sugar. I used G.E.M. Therapy to discover what was contributing to this belief that unless I had sugar I wasn't safe. I processed that issue, and when I completed the process I went back and checked how I was with all the other statements and they were all OK. My craving for sugar stopped, and I was no longer needing sugar all day long. A couple of weeks later I got a call from my son who lives in another state. His words were, "Mom have you been messing with me?" He was asking if I had done energy work on him. I assured him that I was not. When I inquired as to why he asked he told me that he had gone out with his friend for a beer and every time he took a drink it tasted like crap to him. I then told him about my experience of needing sugar to feel safe. My daughter had a similar experience with her craving for sour cream, butter and cheese on mashed potatoes. That combination was comfort food for her. She shared with me one day she couldn't stand that combination any longer because it was too rich and made her sick. When we compared notes, these experiences coincided with the time I was working on the generational issues with sugar. I found it interesting that there is alcohol abuse on both sides of my family, that we were all being affected by "needing sugar to feel safe," but we were using different things to sooth that negative energy.

Chapter 5

Master List Of Essentials Oils

*T*his list of oils will allow you to process all the oils listed in the book without having to flip pages back and forth. The columns allow for efficient processing.

Columns 1–3 are Single Oils

COLUMN 1	COLUMN 2	COLUMN 3
1. Arborvitae	1. Coriander	1. Juniper Berry
2. Basil	2. Cypress	2. Kumquat
3. Bergamot	3. Dill	3. Lavender
4. Birch	4. Douglas Fir	4. Lemon
5. BK Pepper	5. Eucalyptus	5. Lemongrass
6. Cardamom	6. Fennel	6. Lime
7. Cassia	7. Frankincense	7. Marjoram
8. Cedarwood	8. Geranium	8. Melaleuca
9. Cilantro	9. Ginger	9. Melissa
10. Cinnamon	10. Grapefruit	10. Myrrh
11. Clary Sage	11. H. Sandalwood	11. Oregano
12. Clove	12. Helichrysum	12. Patchouli
13. Cumin	13. Jasmine	13. Peppermint

Columns 4 and 6 contain Blends

COLUMN 4	COLUMN 5	COLUMN 6
1. Petitgrain	1. Ylang Ylang	1. Metabolic Blend
2. Red Mandarin	2. Anti-Aging Blend	2. Monthly Blend
3. Roman Chamomile	3. Cellular Blend	3. Protective Blend
4. Rose	4. Comforting Blend	4. Repellent Blend
5. Rosemary	5. Cleansing Blend	5. Reassuring Blend
6. Sandalwood	6. Detoxification Blend	6. Restful Blend
7. Spearmint	7. Digestive Blend	7. Renewal Blend
8. Spikenard	8. Encourage Blend	8. Respiratory Blend
9. Tangerine	9. Focus Blend	9. Skin Blend
10. Thyme	10. Grounding Blend	10. Soothing Blend
11. Vetiver	11. Inspiring Blend	11. Sunny Blend
12. White Fir	12. Invigorating Blend	12. Tension Blend
13. Wild Orange	13. Joyful Blend	13. Women's Blend
14. Wintergreen	14. Massage Blend	14. Uplifting Blend

Chapter 6

Making Your Own Blends

When I complete a processing protocol with essential oils I will have the client affirm if they need to have a supporting personal blend to be used over the ensuing week or so. Most companies that sell essential oils have pre-made blends that are very nice and effective; however, there are times when you need to make a personal blend. The process for finding the oils for your blend is very simple with body testing. You can create a blend for any condition, whether mental, emotional, or physical. I have made personal blends for my grandchildren when they were having nightmares. They weren't affirming for any of the single oils or the pre-made blends. The personal blend I made for them did the trick.

Below is a description of the essential oil classifications and how they complement one another. Each classification of oils are in 3 columns, which allows you to quickly "test" which oil is needed. To process each category, your statement will be, "The oil in this category is in Column 1, 2, or 3." When you identify the column, you will then process the oils in that column to determine the oil for that classification. Do that for each of the classifications.

When creating a therapeutic essential oil blend, put 1 ½ teaspoon of carrier oil in a 5 ml roller bottle. To this bottle you will add the number of drops for the 4 classifications, topping off with another 1 ½ teaspoon of your carrier oil. I prefer fractionated coconut oil for my carrier oil as it is clean, light in smell, absorbs quickly and isn't greasy. If you have another carrier oil that you like or have on hand, you can use that. I have used olive oil with success, though it is heavier. I prefer roller bottles to put my blends in. However, you can mix them in any container that has a lid. Store your creations in dark-colored glass bottles. The preference for a dark glass bottle is to keep the light from breaking down the oils over time. It is important to use your oil blend often if acute symptoms are being expressed. My rule of thumb is to apply three times a day or according to how often you have mental, emotional or physical symptoms surfacing. The discomfort would be an indication that the body has metabolized the oils and is in need of another application. You will never use too much, but you can use too little. The key is to stay attuned to your body, and affirm, if and how much you need when you feel your symptoms expressing.

Example of Personal Blends

Make a blend following these statements:

1. "The # 1 **Personifier** for this blend is in column 1, 2, or 3 (**column 2**)

   "The oil is _____." (Affirm the number, **#5 Roman Chamomile**)

Personifier: 2 drops of Roman Chamomile ~ emotions: purposeless, disheartened, drudgery, frustration

2. "The # 1 **Enhancer** for this blend is in column 1, 2, or 3 (**column 3**)

   "The oil is_____. (Affirm the number, **#3 Melissa**)

   Enhancer: 18 drops of Melissa ~ emotions: depression, darkness, suicidal, overwhelmed

3. "The #1 **Equalizer** for this blend is in column 1, 2, or 3 (**column 1**)

   "The oil is _____." (Affirm the number, **#9 Frankincense**)

   Equalizer: 3 drops of Frankincense ~ emotions: spiritually disconnected, distant from father, unprotected, spiritual darkness

4. "The #1 **Modifier** for this oil is in column 1, 2, or 3 (**column 3**)

   "The oil is _____." (Affirm the number, **#3 Tangerine**)

   Modifier: 2 drops of Tangerine ~ overburdened by responsibilities, downtrodden, heavyhearted, lack of joy

Chapter 7

Essential Oil Classifications

#1. Personifier *(1–5% of the blend; 1.4–2.24 drops)*

Oils have very sharp, strong, and long-lasting fragrances. They also have dominant properties with strong therapeutic action.

1. Birch	1. Ginger	1. Rose
2. Cardamom	2. H. Sandalwood	2. Spearmint
3. Cassia	3. Helichrysum	3. Tangerine
4. Cinnamon	4. Patchouli	4. Wild Orange
5. Clary Sage	5. Peppermint	5. Wintergreen
6. Clove	6. Petitgrain	6. Ylang Ylang
7. Coriander	7. Roman Chamomile	

#2. The Enhancer *(50–80% of the blend; 14–22.4 drops)*

Oil should be the predominant oil of the blend as it serves to enhance the properties of the other oils.. Its fragrance is not as sharp as that of the personifier oils and is usually of a shorter duration.

1. Arbovitae	1. Frankincense	1. Melissa
2. Basil	2. Geranium	2. Oregano
3. Bergamot	3. Grapefruit	3. Patchouli
4. Birch	4. Jasmine	4. Petitgrain
5. Cassia	5. Lavender	5. Roman Chamomile
6. Cedarwood	6. Lemon	6. Rose
7. Cilantro	7. Lemongrass	7. Rosemary
8. Cumin	8. Lime	8. Thyme
9. Dill	9. Marjoram	9. Wild Orange
10. Eucalyptus	10. Melaleuca	10. Wintergreen

#3. *Equalizer* (10–15% of the blend; 2.8–4.2 drops)

Oils create balance and synergy among the oils contained in the blend. Their fragrance is also not as sharp as that of the personifier oils and is of a shorter duration.

1. Arbovitae	1. Ginger	1. Myrrh
2. Basil	2. Jasmine	2. Oregano
3. Birch	3. Juniper Berry	3. Red Mandarin
4. Bergamot	4. Kumquat	4. Roman Chamomile
5. Cedarwood	5. Lavender	5. Rose
6. Cypress	6. Lemongrass	6. Sandalwood
7. Douglas Fir	7. Lime	7. Spikenard
8. Fennel	8. Marjoram	8. Thyme
9. Frankincense	9. Melaleuca	9. Vetiver
10. Geranium	10. Melissa	

#4. Modifier *(5–8% of the blend; 1.4–2.24 drops)*

Oils have a mild and short-lived fragrance. These oils add harmony to the blend.

1. Bergamot	1. Hawaiian Sandalwood	1. Petitgrain
2. Cardamom	2. Jasmine	2. Rose
3. Coriander	3. Lavender	3. Sandalwood
4. Eucalyptus	4. Lemon	4. Tangerine
5. Fennel	5. Melissa	5. Ylang Ylang
6. Grapefruit	6. Myrrh	

Chapter 8

Single Oils

*T*he affirmations are written in first person so that they can be inserted into the Renewal Script. When you are reading the Renewal Script, remember you are calling on the different aspects of self to reprogram the subconscious from a negative to a positive.

Arbovitae

Assists my emotional balance and improves my spiritual awareness and meditation.

Emotions being addressed:

1. Ungratefulness
2. Insignificance
3. Pessimism
4. Self-consciousness

Companion Oils:

1. Birch
2. Cedarwood
3. Cassia
4. Eucalyptus

Blend Classification:

Enhancer & Equalizer

Blends with:

1. Birch
2. Cedarwood
3. Cassia
4. Eucalyptus

Basil

Helps me have an open mind and increases clarity of thought. It helps to bring natural renewal to my body.

Emotions Addressed:

1. Overwhelmed
2. Tired
3. Drained
4. Exhausted

Companion Oils:

1. Peppermint
2. Lavender

Blend Classification:

Enhancer & Equalizer

Blends With:

1. Bergamot
2. White fir
3. Helichrysum
4. Lemongrass

1. Cypress
2. Geranium
3. Wintergreen
4. Marjoram

Bergamot

Uplifts and refreshes, bringing hope and courage to love myself without judgment.

Emotions Addressed:

1. Despair
2. Unlovable
3. Hopelessness
4. Unsafe

Companion Oils:

1. Lemon
2. Cassia
3. Melissa

Blend Classification:

Enhancer, Equalizer & Modifier

Blends With:

1. Cypress
2. Eucalyptus
3. Geranium
4. Lavender
5. Ylang Ylang

Birch

Helps me be open to heal ancestral negative patterns, knowing there is support in doing so.

Emotions Addressed:

1. Unsupported
2. Alienation
3. Fear
4. Weak-willed
5. Being too flexible

Companion Oils:

1. White Fir
2. Wintergreen

Blend Classification:

Personifier & Enhancer

Blends With:

1. Basil
2. Cypress
3. Lavender
4. Marjoram

1. Bergamot
2. Geranium
3. Lemongrass
4. Peppermint

Black Pepper

Helps to strengthen my inner courage to reveal my true self, freeing me to express authentically.

Emotions Address:

1. Dishonesty
2. Feeling Trapped
3. Superficiality
4. Feeling Accused

Companion Oils:

1. Vetiver
2. Frankincense
3. Cinnamon
4. Lavender

Blend Classification:

Enhancer

Blends With:

1. Bergamot
2. Clary Sage
3. Clove
4. Frankincense
5. Geranium
6. Lavender
7. Juniper
8. Sandalwood

Cardamom

Assists with confusion. It is uplifting, refreshing and invigorating.

Emotions Addressed:

1. Feeling muddled
2. Feeling a lack of understanding
3. Avoidance
4. Feeling a lack of energy

Companion Oils:

1. Rosemary
2. Frankincense
3. Geranium
4. Lime

Blend Classification:

Equalizer

Blends With:

1. Bergamot
2. Cedarwood
3. Cinnamon
4. Clove
5. Orange
6. Rose
7. Ylang Ylang

Cassia

Brings courage to the shy and timid, helping to see my worth.

Emotions Addressed:

1. Wanting to hide
2. Fearfulness
3. Insecurity
4. Worthlessness

Companion Oils:

1. Clove
2. Bergamot
3. Lavender
4. Melissa

Blend Classification:

Personifier & Enhancer

Blends With:

1. Black Pepper
2. Roman Chamomile
3. Coriander
4. Frankincense
4. Ginger
5. Geranium
6. Rosemary

Cedarwood

Inspires the feeling of community, allowing giving and receiving to and from family and friends.

Emotions Addressed:

1. Loneliness
2. Disconnected
3. Antisocial
4. Pitiful

Companion Oils:

1. Marjoram
2. Birch
3. White Fir

Blend Classification:

Enhancer & Equalizer

Blends With:

1. Bergamot
2. Clary Sage
3. Cypress
4. Eucalyptus
5. Juniper
6. Rosemary

Cilantro

Brings light to my body, heart and soul by releasing the need to control.

Emotions Addressed:

1. Toxic
2. Constricted
3. Obsessiveness
4. Clingy

Companion Oils:

1. Coriander
2. Thyme
3. Cypress

Blend Classification:

Enhancer

Blends With:

1. Bergamot
2. Cinnamon
3. Frankincense
4. Lime
5. Sandalwood

Cinnamon

Which fosters feelings of love and respect for myself and others.

Emotions Addressed:

1. Jealousy
2. Sexual abuse
3. Sexual repression
4. Fearfulness

Companion Oils:

1. Grapefruit
2. Black Pepper
3. Cilantro
4. Patchouli
5. Cilantro

Blend Classification:

Personifier

Blends With:

1. All Citrus Oils
2. Cypress
3. Frankincense
4. Geranium
5. Lavender
6. Rosemary
7. All Spice Oils

Clary Sage

Allows me to recognize incorrect perceptions and to have the courage to make a course correction based on truth.

Emotions Addressed:

1. Confusion
2. Darkness
3. Discouragement
4. Hopelessness

Companion Oils:

1. Lemongrass
2. Black Pepper
3. Melissa
4. Frankincense

Blend Classification:

Personifier

Blends With:

1. Bergamot
2. Citrus Oils
3. Cypress
4. Geranium
5. Sandalwood

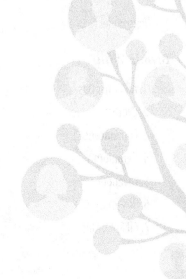

Clove

Helps me to feel protected and have the courage to overcome a victim mentality.

Emotions Addressed:

1. Victimization
2. Defeated
3. Feeling dominated
4. Feeling enslaved

Companion Oils:

1. Ginger
2. Birch
3. Black Pepper
4. Melaleuca

Blend Classification:

Personifier

Blends With:

1. Basil	1. Bergamot
2. Cinnamon	2. Clary Sage
3. Grapefruit	3. Lavender
4. Lemon	4. Orange
5. Peppermint	5. Rose
6. Rosemary	6. Ylang Ylang

Coriander

Enables me to be loyal to myself. Seeing my self-worth fosters the ability to be true to myself.

Emotions Addressed:

1. Feeling controlled by others
2. Self-betrayal
3. Drudgery
4. Instability

Companion Oils:

1. Frankincense
2. Cilantro
3. Lavender
4. Roman Chamomile

Blend Classification:

Personifier & Modifier

Blends With:

1. Bergamot
2. Cinnamon
3. Clary Sage
4. Cypress
5. Ginger
6. Sandalwood
7. Spice

Cumin

Fills me with wisdom, which is pure, peaceable, and full of mercy.

Emotions Addressed:

1. Unhappiness
2. Sorrowfulness
3. Feeling distressed
4. Uncomfortableness

Companion Oils:

1. Dill
2. Fennel
3. Peppermint

Blend Classification:

Enhancer

Blends With:

1. Cilantro
2. Coriander
3. Wintergreen
4. Frankincense

Cypress

Enables me to let go of the past and flow with the joy of the present.

Emotions Addressed:

1. Feeling controlling
2. Perfectionism
3. Rigidity
4. Feeling tense

Companion Oils:

1. Peppermint
2. Cilantro
3. Vetiver
4. Thyme

Blend Classification:

Equalizer

Blends With:

1. Lemon
2. Lime
3. Grapefruit
4. Wild Orange
5. Bergamot

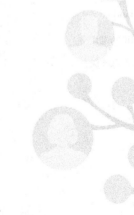

Dill

Redirects my fear into faith.

Emotions Addressed:

1. Nervousness
2. Fidgety
3. Feeling restricted
4. Jittery

Companion Oils:

1. Bergamot
2. All Citrus Oils

Blend Classification:

Enhancer

Blends With:

1. All Citrus Oils

Douglas Fir:

Elevates and stabilizes my mind and emotions with hope.

Emotions Addressed:

1. Feeling frazzled
2. Feeling a lack of understanding
3. Not cherished
4. Unable to flow with life

Classification:

Equalizer

Companion Oils:

1. White Fir
2. Frankincense
3. Clary Sage
4. Sandalwood

Blends With:

1. Cedarwood
2. Eucalyptus
3. Frankincense
4. Juniper Berry
5. Peppermint
6. Rosemary

Eucalyptus

Which relieves the need to be ill, allowing healing to happen on the emotional and spiritual level.

Emotions Address:

1. Attachment to illness
2. Clinginess
3. Desire to escape life
4. Putting off responsibilities

Companion Oils:

1. Helichrysum

Blend Classification:

Enhancer

Blends With:

1. Ginger
2. Lemon
3. Melaleuca
4. Rosemary

Fennel

Provides support when I have a weakened sense of self. This increased self-awareness nourishes my body and soul.

Emotions Addressed:

1. Lack of desire
2. Shame
3. Weakness
4. Unfeeling

Companions Oils:

1. Sandalwood
2. Grapefruit
3. Ginger

Blend Classification:

Equalizer & Modifier

Blends With:

1. Basil
2. Geranium
3. Lavender
4. Lemon
5. Rosemary

Frankincense

Assists me in letting go of lower vibrations, lies, deceptions and negativity and inviting the light of the divine to bring healing.

Emotions Addressed:

1. Feeling spiritually disconnected
2. Feeling distant from father
3. Feeling unprotected
4. Spiritual darkness

Companion Oils:

1. Myrrh
2. Roman Chamomile
3. Clary Sage
4. Melissa

Blend Classification:

Enhancer & Equalizer

Blends With:

All Oils

Geranium

Restores confidence in the goodness of others; helps heal my broken heart.

Emotions Addressed:

1. Abandonment
2. Loss
3. Distrustfulness
4. Feeling disheartened

Companion Oils:

1. Marjoram
2. Ylang Ylang
3. Rose

Blend Classification:

Enhancer & Equalizer

Blends With:

All Oils

Ginger

Enables me to be fully present, to take responsibility and let go of being a victim.

Emotions Addressed:

1. Feeling like a victim
2. Powerlessness
3. Defeatedness
4. Blaming

Companion Oils:

1. Clove
2. Fennel
3. Helichrysum
4. Melaleuca

Blend Classification:

Personifier & Equalizer

Blends With:

1. All Spice Oils
2. All Citrus Oils
3. Eucalyptus
4. Frankincense
5. Geranium
6. Rosemary

Grapefruit

Encourages a feeling of respect & love for my body.

Emotions Addressed:

1. Hate for the body
2. Addiction to food
3. Eating disorder
4. Anxiety over appearance

Companion Oils:

1. Patchouli
2. Fennel
3. Rosemary

Blend Classification:

Enhancer & Modifier

Blends With:

1. Basil
2. Bergamot
3. Cypress
4. Frankincense
5. Geranium
6. Lavender
7. Peppermint
8. Ylang Ylang

Hawaiian Sandalwood

Assists in quieting my mind to hear the subtle whispering of the spirit

Emotions Addressed:

1. Fearful
2. Numb
3. Nervous
4. Hopeless

Companion Oils:

1. Oregano
2. Frankincense
3. Myrrh

Blend Classification:

Personifier & Modifier

Blends With:

1. Cypress
2. Frankincense
3. Lemon
4. Myrrh
5. Ylang Ylang

Helichrysum

Removes pain quickly and effortlessly, aiding "the walking wounded."

Emotions Addressed:

1. Intense pain
2. Anguish
3. Turmoil
4. Wounded

Companion Oils:

1. Ginger
2. Wintergreen

Blend Classification:

Personifier

Blends With:

1. Geranium
2. Clary Sage
3. Rose
4. Lavender
5. Spice Oils
6. Citrus Oils

Jasmine

Increases intuitive powers inviting wisdom, and inviting inspirational relationships.

Emotions Addressed:

1. Feeling low
2. Feeling disrespected
3. Uncomfortableness [or Discomfort]
4. Feeling unkind

Companion Oils:

1. Helichrysum
2. Wild Orange

Blend Classification:

Enhancer, Equalizer & Modifier

Blends With:

1. Bergamot
2. Frankincense
3. Geranium
4. Helichrysum
5. Lemongrass
6. Melissa
7. Wild Orange
8. Rose
9. Sandalwood
10. Spearmint

Juniper Berry

Brings light into the dark and hidden aspects of myself.

Emotions Addressed:

1. Irrational fears
2. Recurrent nightmares
3. Restless sleep
4. Helplessness

Companion Oils:

1. Black Pepper
2. Clary Sage
3. Vetiver

Blend Classification:

Equalizer

Blends With:

1. Bergamot
2. All Citrus Oils
3. Cypress
4. Geranium
5. Lavender
6. Melaleuca
7. Rosemary

Kumquat

Invites love to revitalize and refresh my mind.

Emotions Addressed:

1. Insecurity
2. Jitteriness
3. Superficiality
4. Discontentedness

Companion Oils:

1. Lemon
2. Lime
3. Wild Orange
4. Bergamot

Blend Classification:

Equalizer

Blends With:

1. Clove
2. Lavender
3. Patchouli
4. Roman Chamomile

Lavender

Connects my heart and soul allowing for better communication.

Emotions Addressed:

1. Fear of rejection
2. Constricted
3. Tension
4. Wanting to hide

Companion Oils:

1. Lime
2. Cassia

Blend Classification:

Enhancer, Equalizer & Modifier

Blends With:

1. Wild Orange
2. Lemon
3. Grapefruit
4. Clary Sage
5. Geranium

Lemon

Enables my focus to be present, inviting feelings of happiness and joy, fostering confidence in my abilities.

Emotions Addressed:

1. Confusion
2. Inability to focus
3. Mental fatigue
4. Lack of energy
5. Learning disorders

Companion Oils:

1. Rosemary
2. Peppermint

Blend Classification:

Enhancer & Modifier

Blends With:

1. Eucalyptus
2. Fennel
3. Frankincense
4. Geranium
5. Sandalwood
6. Ylang Ylang

Lemongrass

Initiates cleansing and healing in all aspects of my being.

Emotions Addressed:

1. Negative energy
2. Despair
3. Darkness
4. Spiritual blindness

Companion Oils:

1. Melaleuca
2. Thyme
3. Clary Sage
4. Geranium

Blend Classification:

Enhancer & Equalizer

Blends With:

1. Basil
2. Clary Sage
3. Eucalyptus
4. Lavender
5. Melaleuca
6. Rosemary

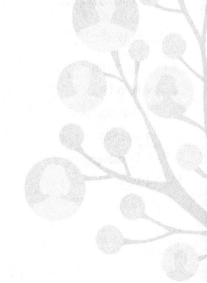

Lime

Assists me to have the courage to feel from the heart.

Emotions Addressed:

1. Apathy
2. Resignation
3. Grief
4. Suicidal ideation

Companion Oils:

1. Tangerine
2. Lavender

Blend Classification:

Enhancer & Equalizer

Blends With:

1. Bergamot
2. Cypress
3. Wild Orange
4. Rosemary
5. Ylang Ylang

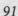

Marjoram

Invites trust to heal my heart from old wounds, restoring and establishing true bonds of love and friendship.

Emotions Addressed:

1. Distrust
2. Aloofness
3. Feeling distant
4. Emotional isolation

Companion Oils:

1. Cedarwood
2. Rosemary
3. Geranium

Blend Classification:

Enhancer & Equalizer

Blends With:

1. Bergamot
2. Cypress
3. Lavender
4. Wild Orange
5. Rosemary
6. Ylang Ylang

Melaleuca

Enables me to recognize incorrect perceptions that allowed toxic relationships to exist.

Emotions Addressed:

1. Codependency
2. No Boundaries
3. Weak-willed
4. Lack of self-confidence

Companion Oils:

1. Thyme
2. Lemongrass
3. Purify

Blend Classification:

Enhancer & Equalizer

Blends With:

1. All Citrus Oils
2. Cypress
3. Eucalyptus
4. Lavender
5. Rosemary
6. Thyme

Melissa

Floods my being with the joy of living.

Emotions Addressed:

1. Depression
2. Darkness
3. Suicidal ideation
4. Feeling overwhelmed

Companion Oils:

1. Lime
2. Tangerine

Blend Classification:

Enhancer, Equalizer & Modifier

Blends With:

1. Geranium
2. Lavender
3. Jasmine
4. Wild Orange
5. Rose
6. Ylang Ylang

Myrrh

Invites feeling of trust and safety from a nurturing feminine energy.

Emotions Addressed:

1. Unhappiness
2. Wounded
3. Imbalanced
4. Feeling dishonored

Companion Oils:

1. Clary Sage
2. Frankincense

Blend Classification:

Equalizer & Modifier

Blends With:

1. Frankincense
2. Lavender
3. Sandalwood
4. Black Pepper

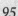

Oregano

Invites the soul to be one with God, encourages letting go of limiting beliefs and relationships.

Emotions Addressed:

1. Being opinionated
2. Negativity
3. Uncomfortableness [or Discomfort]
4. Feeling lack of support

Companion Oils:

1. Sandalwood
2. Thyme
3. Melaleuca
4. Lemongrass

Blend Classification:

Enhancer & Equalizer

Blends With:

1. Basil
2. Fennel
3. Geranium
4. Lemongrass
5. Thyme
6. Rosemary

Patchouli

Encourages me to be present on the deepest level with my physical body, inviting a oneness between the spirit and physical body.

Emotions Addressed:

1. Body shame
2. Judgment of the body
3. Lack of concern for self
4. Body tension

Companion Oils:

1. Grapefruit
2. Cinnamon

Blend Classification:

Enhancer

Blends With:

1. Bergamot
2. Frankincense
3. Ginger
4. Lemongrass
5. Pine
6. Sandalwood

1. Clary Sage
2. Geranium
3. Lavender
4. Myrrh
5. Rosewood

Peppermint

Enables my heart to view pain as a valuable teacher, bringing buoyancy to my heart.

Emotions Addressed:

1. Unbearable pain
2. Intense depression
3. Heaviness
4. Avoidance

Companion Oils:

1. Tangerine
2. Lime
3. Rose
4. Cypress

Blend Classification:

Personifier

Blends With:

1. Rosemary
2. Black Pepper
3. Eucalyptus
4. Geranium
5. Melaleuca

Petitgrain

Assists me to serve others with reverence and awe.

Emotions Addressed:

1. Shock
2. Fear
3. Sleeplessness
4. Anger

Companion Oils:

1. Lavender
2. Sandalwood
3. Bergamot

Blend Classification:

Enhancer and Modifier

Blends With:

1. Cassia
2. Cinnamon
3. Geranium

Red Mandarin

Brings comfort and support to my whole spirit, soul, and body.

Emotions Addressed:

1. Feeling burdened
2. Feeling dreary
3. Purposelessness
4. Feeling worthless

Companion Oils:

1. Lemon
2. Lime
3. Wild Orange
4. Grapefruit

Blend Classification:

Equalizer

Blends With:

1. Clove
2. Cinnamon
3. Bergamot
4. Frankincense
5. Lavender

Roman Chamomile

Helps me to not feel alone as I follows my spiritual path. Bringing contentment and direction to my purpose and mission.

Emotions Addressed:

1. Purposelessness
2. Feeling disheartened
3. Drudgery
4. Frustration

Companion Oil:

1. Frankincense
2. Melissa

Blend Classification:

Personifier

Blends With:

1. Lavender
2. Rose
3. Geranium
4. Clary Sage

Rose

Draws my heart to divine love, helping me to remember the healing power that it brings.

Emotions Addressed:

1. Feeling bereft of divine love
2. Having constricted feelings
3. Having a closed heart
4. Feeling a lack of love

Companion Oils:

1. Geranium
2. Ylang Ylang
3. Thyme
4. Clary Sage

Blend Classification:

Personifier, Enhancer, Equalizer & Modifier

Blends With:

All Oils

Rosemary

Assists me to reach deep within to find true knowledge.

Emotions Addressed:

1. Confusion
2. Difficulty in adjusting
3. Difficulty in transitioning
4. Difficulty in learning

Companion Oils:

1. Lemon
2. Marjoram

Blend Classification:

Enhancer

Blend With:

1. Basil
2. Frankincense
3. Lavender
4. Peppermint
5. Eucalyptus

Sandalwood

Invites my mind and heart to quiet, centering on the knowledge that humility, devotion, and love are divine qualities.

Emotions Addressed:

1. Unable to feel God
2. Disconnected from self
3. Emptiness
4. Overthinking

Companion Oils:

1. Oregano
2. Frankincense

Blend Classification:

Equalizer & Modifier

Blends With:

1. Cypress
2. Frankincense
3. Lemon
4. Myrrh
5. Ylang Ylang

Spearmint

Helps me to access inner light, allowing me to share that light with clarity and confidence.

Emotions Addressed:

1. Fear of expressing opinions
2. Shyness
3. Timidity
4. Fear of public speaking

Companion Oils:

1. Cassia
2. Lavender

Blend Classification:

Personifier

Blends With:

1. Basil
2. Lavender
3. Peppermint
4. Rosemary

Spikenard

Invites a calm and relaxed state of patience while I am being perfected.

Emotions Addressed:

1. Furious
2. Phony
3. Panic
4. Irresponsibility

Companion Oils:

1. Lavender
2. Myrrh
3. Clary Sage

Blend Classification:

Equalizer

Blends With:

1. Frankincense
2. Lavender
3. Wild Orange
4. Petitgrain
5. Rose

Tangerine

Assists me to recognize my natural creativity, allowing me to invite the joyful and playful child spirit to return.

Emotions Addressed:

1. Feeling overburdened by responsibilities
2. Feeling downtrodden
3. Heavyheartedness
4. Lack of joy

Companion Oils:

1. Wild Orange
2. Ylang Ylang
3. Roman Chamomile
4. Lime

Blend Classification:

Personifier & Modifier

Blends With:

1. Basil
2. Clary Sage
3. Geranium
4. Lavender
5. Wild Orange

1. Bergamot
2. Frankincense
3. Grapefruit
4. Lemon
5. Roman Chamomile

Thyme

Assists in releasing negative feelings and thoughts from my heart, making room for love and forgiveness.

Emotions Addressing:

1. Having an unforgiving heart
2. Anger
3. Rage
4. Bitterness

Companion Oils:

1. Cypress
2. Lemongrass

Blend Classification:

Enhancer& Equalizer

Blends With:

1. Bergamot
2. Melaleuca
3. Oregano
4. Rosemary

Vetiver

Keeps me in the present while working through deep-rooted emotions to reveal my true self.

Emotions Addressed:

1. Apathetic
2. Despondence
3. Feeling scattered
4. Feeling stressed

Companion Oils:

1. Black Pepper
2. Cypress

Blend Classification:

Equalizer

Blends With:

1. Clary Sage
2. Lavender
3. Rose
4. Sandalwood
5. Ylang Ylang

White Fir

Awakens healing that comes to the heart, mind, body, and soul when I am willing to address generational issues.

Emotions Addressed:

1. Feeling overburdened
2. Having unidentified fears
3. Addictions
4. Abuse

Companion Oils:

1. Birch
2. Cedarwood

Blend Classification:

Equalizer

Blends With:

1. Frankincense
2. Lavender

Wild Orange

Encourages the recognition that abundance is a divine gift extended to all, calling forth childlike qualities of freedom and claiming all that life offers.

Emotions Addressed:

1. Scarcity
2. Feeling overly serious
3. Negativity
4. Feeling a lack of opportunities

Companion Oils:

1. Tangerine
2. Ylang Ylang
3. Lemon
4. Peppermint

Blend Classification:

Personifier, Enhancer

Blends With:

1. Cinnamon
2. Frankincense
3. Geranium
4. Lavender

Wintergreen

Encourages me to let go and allow spiritual healing and resolution.

Emotions Addressed:

1. Needing to control
2. Willfulness
3. Prideful
4. Opinionated

Companion Oils:

1. Sandalwood
2. Oregano
3. Birch
4. Eucalyptus
5. Frankincense

Blend Classification:

Personifier & Enhancer

Blends With:

1. Basil
2. Bergamot
3. Cypress
4. Geranium
5. Lavender
6. Lemongrass
7. Marjoram
8. Peppermint

Ylang Ylang

Helps release addictions and emotional trauma from my heart.

Emotions Addressed:

1. Feeling overstressed
2. Grief
3. Sadness
4. Feeling uptight

Companion Oils:

1. Tangerine
2. Wild Orange
3. Rose
4. Geranium

Blend Classification:

Personifier & Modifier

Blends With:

1. Bergamot
2. Geranium
3. Grapefruit
4. Lemon
5. Marjoram
6. Sandalwood
7. Vetiver

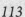

Chapter 9

Oil Blends

Anti-Aging Blend

Aids in quieting my mind, inviting inner stillness and spiritual growth.

Emotions Addressed:

1. Darkness
2. Spiritual blindness
3. Feeling burdened
4. Feeling discouraged

Companion Oils:

1. Frankincense
2. Sandalwood
3. Wintergreen
4. Helichrysum
5. Rose

Cellular Blend

Assists me in reclaiming my health, embracing the cycle of life and rebirth.

Emotions Addressed:

1. Weariness
2. Feeling disheartened
3. Feeling stuck in old family patterns

Companion Oils:

1. Eucalyptus
2. Frankincense
3. Basil

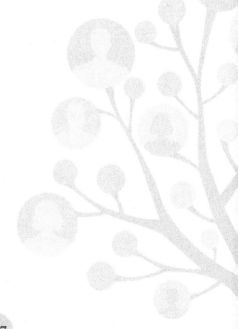

Cleansing Blend

Aids in purification of old thoughts, allowing a continual flow of the new ideas.

Emotions Addressed:

1. Feeling unable to let go
2. Inability to move forward
3. Negative emotions

Companion Oils:

1. Lemongrass
2. Thyme
3. Cilantro

Comforting Blend

Helps to ease my grief to invite calm, peace, and happiness to enter my life.

Emotions Addressed:

1. Grief
2. Sadness
3. Hopelessness
4. Feeling persecuted

Companion Oils:

1. Geranium
2. Lime
3. Peppermint

Detoxification Blend

Assists in letting go of the old toxic beliefs and habits that keep me stuck.

Emotions Addressed:

1. Unwillingness to transition
2. Addiction
3. Incorrect perceptions

Companion Oils:

1. Lemongrass
2. Rosemary
3. Melaleuca
4. Clove
5. Cilantro

Digestive Blend

Helps me to digest and assimilate new experiences.

Emotions Addressed:

1. Loss of appetite for life
2. Inability to assimilate new experiences
3. Feeling overwhelmed

Companion Oils:

1. Rosemary
2. Fennel
3. Ginger
4. Lemon

Encouraging Blend

Calls forth confidence and courage, to trust myself knowing I am not alone.

Emotions Addressed:

1. Doubt
2. Pessimism
3. Cynicism
4. Lack of trust

Companion Oils:

1. Wild Orange
2. Tangerine
3. Peppermint
4. Myrrh

Focus Blend

Calms my mind, facilitating inner peace and the ability to stay in the present.

Emotions Addressed:

1. Interference
2. Lack of physical presence
3. Lack of awareness
4. Feeling scattered

Companion Oils:

1. Patchouli
2. Sandalwood
3. Vetiver

Grounding Blend

Helps me to stay grounded and see my vision manifested.

Emotions Addressed:

1. Feeling scattered
2. Disconnectedness
3. Lack of stability
4. Feeling unable to be responsible

Companion Oils:

1. Birch
2. Myrrh
3. Patchouli
4. Vetiver

Inspiring Blend

Facilitates letting go of fear and acting with inspiration and passion.

Emotions Addressed:

1. Apathy
2. Lack of interest
3. Indifference
4. Lack of creativity

Companion Oils:

1. Vetiver
2. Tangerine
3. Lavender

Invigorating Blend

Strengthens and reinforces my motivation and drive when it is lacking.

Emotions Addressed:

1. Stifled creativity
2. Blocked creativity
3. Fear of self-expression
4. Feeling emotionally imbalanced
5. Low will to live

Companion Oils:

1. Tangerine
2. Wild Orange
3. Joyful Blend

Joyful Blend

Allows me to choose being happy, carefree and living an abundant life.

Emotions Addressed:

1. Low energy
2. Depression
3. Darkness
4. Seriousness
5. Sternness

Companion Oils:

1. Tangerine
2. Melissa
3. Ylang Ylang
4. Wild Orange

Massage Blend

Allows my heart to open to life and living as my body relaxes.

Emotions Addressed:

1. Stiffness in body
2. Stiffness in mind
3. Stressed

Companion Oils:

1. Cypress
2. Basil
3. Peppermint

Metabolic Blend

Allows my body to release emotional pounds.

Emotions Addressed:

1. Disgust of physical body
2. Feeling ugly
3. Feeling of worthlessness

Companion Oils:

1. Grapefruit
2. Cinnamon
3. Patchouli
4. Bergamot

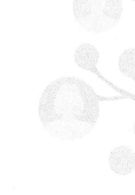

Monthly Blend

Encourages me to embrace my gender with confidence and joy.

Emotions Addressed:

1. Vulnerability
2. Closed
3. Dread of menstruation
4. Dread of menopause

Companion Oils:

1. Myrrh
2. Marjoram
3. Geranium
4. Cedarwood
5. Ylang Ylang

Protective Blend

Aids in setting boundaries in relationships.

Emotions Addressed:

1. Feeling unprotected
2. Feeling threatened
3. Vulnerability
4. Giving into peer pressure

Companion Oils:

1. Clove
2. Ginger

Reassuring Blend

Calls me to remember love is forever available to me, and I am never separated from divine love.

Emotions Addressed:

1. Anxiety
2. Fearfulness
3. Worry
4. Stress

Companion Oils:

1. Basil
2. Sandalwood
3. Cypress
4. Myrrh

Renewal Blend

Encourages feelings of safety and love for myself.

Emotions Addressed:

1. Feelings of guilt
2. Feeling unsafe
3. Unloved
4. Mental fatigue

Companion Oils:

1. Cypress
2. Geranium
3. Sandalwood
4. Rosemary

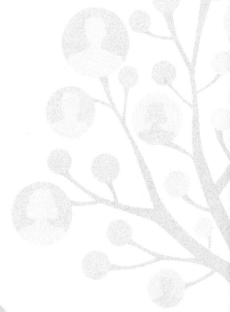

Repellent Blend

Helps me to stay calm in the face of danger or attack.

Emotions Addressed:

1. Feeling unprotected
2. Feeling attacked
3. Defenselessness

Companion Oils:

1. Melaleuca
2. Clove
3. Ginger

Respirtory Blend

Addresses my inability to let go of grief and pain.

Emotions Addressed:

1. Sadness
2. Grief
3. Despair
4. Feeling unloved
5. Distrust

Companion Oils:

1. Lime
2. Eucalyptus
3. White Fir

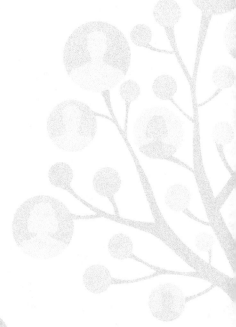

Restful Blend

Allows me to forgive all offenses.

Emotions Addressed:

1. Resentment
2. Inability to forgive
3. Perfectionism
4. Jealousy

Companion Oils:

1. Geranium
2. Marjoram
3. Rose
4. Ylang Ylang

Skin Blend

Invites me to embrace forgiveness of self and others.

Emotions Addressed:

1. Pain
2. Rage
3. Self-judgment

Companion Oils:

1. Bergamot
2. Melissa
3. Cinnamon

Soothing Blend

Aids facing emotional wounds, allowing them to surface and heal.

Emotions Addressed:

1. Resistance to pain
2. Avoiding emotional issues
3. Fear of painful situations

Companion Oils:

1. Helichrysum
2. Wintergreen

Sunny Blend

Assists my heart in opening and receiving the abundant gifts that the universe is offering.

Emotions Addressed:

1. Feeling peeved
2. Feeling Driven
3. Feeling imprisoned
4. Feeling insignificant

Companion Oils:

1. Grapefruit
2. Wild Orange
3. Peppermint

Tension Blend

Helps me find calm, bringing peace to my body, mind, and spirit.

Emotions Addressed:

1. Stress
2. Nervousness
3. Feeling overwhelmed
4. Exhaustion

Companion Oils:

1. Cypress
2. Peppermint
3. Thyme

Uplifting Blend

Brings abundance to my hope and dreams as I stay in the present.

Emotions Addressed:

1. Feeling enslaved
2. Feeling defeated
3. Feeling undervalues
4. Feeling restricted

Companion Oils:

1. Sandalwood
2. Rose
3. Wild Orange

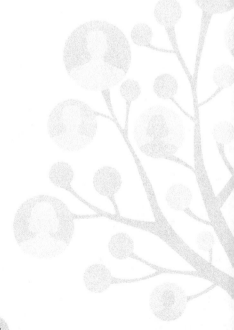

Woman's Blend

Helps me joyfully embrace my feminine energy.

Emotions Addressed:

1. Feeling overly masculine
2. Blocked female energy
3. Irritability
4. Tough exterior

Companion Oils:

1. Myrrh
2. Geranium
3. Ylang Ylang
4. Bergamot

Glossary

Factors:

Factors indicate how we perceive an event, person, action, statement, or the intent behind the action that created the feeling. For example, take the statement, "I am not good enough." The emotion attached to that is going to feel different depending on which of the following factors was at the root of that emotion. If it is based on Evil the emotion is going to be different that if it was created because of an Error of Thought.

1. **Error of Though:** the state or condition of being wrong in conduct or judgment

2. **Negative Emotion:** a statement or decision expressing or implying denial, disagreement, or refusal.

3. **Negative Words:** the feeling being set up based on negative words being used.

4. **Lies:** involving deception or founded on a mistaken impression, presenting a false impression.

5. **Evil:** an action against another with the intent to harm, malign, discredit, shame, etc.

Family:

Mankind has been in units throughout history as we know it. The thought of the author is that if we were spirit children and adults, that perhaps we have always been in the units we find ourselves in as humans.

1. **Universal Family:** All persons born to this earth.

2. **Tribes:** A unit of the Universal Family, indicating the tribe on the father's or mother's side, or both.

3. **Family:** A smaller unit of the tribe, indicating the family on the father's or mother's side, or both

4. **Individual:** self, male or female

Phases:

Phases represent a time and space in which a person has existed based on different beliefs. Some will believe in the creation plan, others will believe in reincarnation, others will believe that we are just part of a universal galaxy existence. I have based "Phases" off the belief that we have existed with a deity figure. You can adjust phases to align with your beliefs. The main thing is to open your mind to the possibility of time and space, however that looks to you. Understand that the opportunity for an incorrect perception to be created in any of these phases, leaves the possibility for it to continue resonating in the energy field that supports us.

1. **Spiritual childhood:** Our beginning, whatever that means to you.

2. **Spiritual adulthood:** Revelations 12:7–8 states, "And there was a war in heaven: Michael and his angels fought against the dragon; and the dragon fought and his angels, and they prevailed not; neither was their place found any more in heaven." Regardless whether you hold this belief, it brings up the possibility of maturity in a spirit state the same as in mortal life.

3. **Creation of the physical body:** In the creation model, the body was created to house the spirit. The physical body has an intelligence separate from the mind.

4. **Integration into physical body:** Indicating a transition state into the physical world that the spirit passes through, gathering information for the journey into the physical.

5. **Earth life:** Having a physical body.

6. **Afterlife:** When something is still an issue for an individual who has passed on to the other side, they will need help releasing an emotion that was set up when in the physical body. It is as if they need someone to feel the emotion to have the negative energy dispersed.

Author's Notes

My hope and prayer is that you will find help and comfort from this book. There are no new feelings, thoughts, and emotions; they are just all recycling and magnifying as they keep passing down through the generations. It is time to stop the madness.

We all have a desire for peace, contentment and fulfillment in our lives. One of the ways we seek that is through prayer. In scripture, we read in Matthew 7:7, which states, "Ask, and it shall be given you, seek and ye shall find, knock and it shall be opened unto you."[1]

In 2 Nephi 32:4, it states, "Wherefore, now after I have spoken these words, if ye cannot understand them it will be because ye asked not, neither do ye knock; wherefore, ye are not brought into the light, but must perish in the dark."[2]

Gregg Braden shared in his book, *The Isaiah Effect*, "The power of prayer is found in a force that cannot be spoken or transmitted as the written word—the *feeling* that the prayer's words evoke within us. It is the feeling of our prayers that opens the door and illuminates our paths to the forces of the seen as well as the unseen." Speaking with a Tibetan abbot, he also learned that "feeling was

---

1 *New Testament, Holy Bible*
2 *Book of Mormon*, Published by The Church of Jesus Christ of Latter-day Saints

more than just a *factor* in prayer. He emphasized that *feeling is the prayer!*"[3]

When we can make a lasting change in our life it is because we *feel* the need for change. If we can go to the root of the problem and identify some generational emotions they will in turn allow us to *feel* what needs to be changed. This allows us to reprogram a negative feeling into a positive feeling.

This process enables us to be specific with words we seek in prayer to heal our body, mind and soul. When we gather the right keys to unlock the door of our hurt, sorrow, anger, loneliness, fear, etc., that invites the divine flow of love, goodness, and abundance, which in turn are at the root of true healing.

I hope your mind has been expanded. Know that this process does not have to be followed exactly. Be open to your own intuition and revelation. Any good teacher wants the student to soar and go beyond to new heights and knowledge. If you already have protocols that work for you, see what parts and pieces of what you have learned here can be added to your own Wellness Tool Box. If you like what you have read here please spread the word. Each time reprogramming is done it changes all of us for the better.

Note To Readers: This book was originally a manual in a 3-ring binder. It is much easier to use the book in the spiral form for processing. You can always take this book to a print store and for a few bucks they will spiral bind it for you.

---

3 Braden, Greg. *The Isaiah Effect.* Three Rivers Press, 2000. Available on Amazon.com.

Reading List

I would like to share a few books that have made a huge difference in my life. Some of them may call to you as well. You will notice that the top four books are religious books. I have found that most of us have religion in our history regardless of whether we espouse it currently. For some of us it will have a positive memory but for others religion was difficult and sometimes harmful and hurtful. If so, those feeling need to be addressed and healed. We all need to look at the way we were raised, embracing the good and the healing, and eliminating the parts that don't serve us in a healthy way. All of these books deal with feeling and emotions in one way or another.

Old and New Testament, any publication

Book of Mormon, Church of Jesus Christ of Latter-day Saints

Doctrine and Covenants, Church of Jesus Christ of Latter-day Saints

The Pearl of Great Price, Church of Jesus Christ of Latter-day Saints

Feelings Buried Alive Never Die, by Karol Truman. Olympus
Distributing, 2003

Healing Feeling from the Heart, by Karol Truman. Olympus
Distributing, 2011

Remembering Wholeness, by Carol Tuttle. Elton-Wolf Publishing,
2002

The Isaiah Effect, by Gregg Braden. Three Rivers Press, *2000*

Awakening to Zero Point, by Gregg Braden. Sacred Spaces/Ancient
Wisdom, 1999

Biology of Belief, by Bruce Lipton. Mountain of Love/Elite Books,
2005

Molecules of Emotion, by Candace B. Pert. Touchstone, 1999

About the Author

Joyce Turkington is the owner of K-Bay Wellness Center. Joyce has lived in Homer, Alaska, most of her life. She married her high school sweetheart, and together with her husband Alan, they raised four children. Joyce's interest in healthcare and wellness coaching came from her own diagnosis of 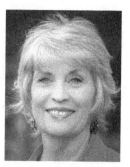 Multiple Sclerosis at age 24. Using different holistic therapies, she has been symptom free for 40 years.

Joyce is a public speaker, teacher, instructor, coach and facilitator. She is an expert in helping others discover the generational emotions that are at the root of their symptoms. She teaches them the art of identifying and eliminating the negative perceptions that have a direct effect on their DNA by inserting the exact words that cleanse and charge the energy field for all generations. Over the past seven years, she has been using essential oils as part of her therapy. Aromatherapy is very effective in assisting to relieve stress.

Contact

For more information about the essential oils the author uses, you can go to her business website. Having a quality essential oil is critical. Remember we are working to raise your vibration. Each essential oil has hertz vibration that can assist in atoning the body. Having a pure oil without fillers is very important. To educate yourself about the purity of essential oils, you might want to check out world-renowned EO chemist Dr. Robert Pappas at **www.essentialoils.org**

Blessings to you and thank you for your interest. You can follow the author at these sites:

www.kbaywellnesscenter.com

www.facebook.com/KBay-Wellness-Center-128316587226987/

If you wish to contact Joyce, you can do so through either of these websites.

9 780999 317808

Printed in March 2021
by Rotomail Italia S.p.A., Vignate (MI) - Italy